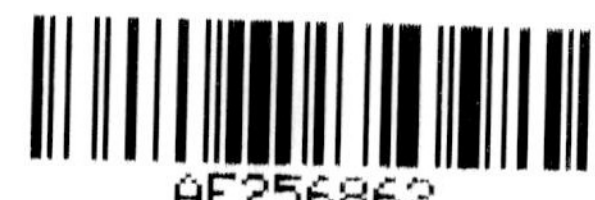

This Book Belongs To:

____

SALAD

SALAD

SALAD